The Outlive And Longevity Diet

For Absolute Beginners

Embrace a Plant-Based Lifestyle for Optimal Health, Increased Energy, and Vibrant Living - A Guide to Reduce Inflammation, Balance Gut Health.

i

TABLE OF CONTENT

INTRODUCTION

People have sought the aim of having a full and healthy life for as long as possible throughout human history. Recent advances in science and medicine have enabled us to dive further into the complexity of aging and the factors that influence the duration of our lives. This chapter attempts to give a comprehensive explanation of longevity by examining the science of aging, the numerous factors that impact the human lifetime, and the major role that nutrition plays in the aging process.

The Science of Aging

Aging, a complex and multifaceted biological process, is defined by a steady decline in physiological performance over time. Aging causes a slew of changes at the cellular level, including the accumulation of damage to cells, a decrease in cells' ability to repair themselves, and changes in gene expression. To understand the science of aging, a deeper examination of these fundamental elements is required.

Cellular aging is closely linked to a decrease in the length of telomeres, which are protective extensions found at the ends of chromosomes. Cells experience cellular senescence, a process in which they lose the ability to divide further due to the gradual shortening of their telomeres, which serve as a biological clock. This contributes to the development of age-related illnesses as well as general tissue function loss.

Furthermore, the importance of mitochondria, the cell's powerhouse, in the aging process cannot be overstated. Mitochondria, an important component of energy production, are susceptible to oxidative stress over time, which can cause damage and eventually reduce their functionality. Reduced mitochondrial activity has been linked to a variety of age-related illnesses, including cardiovascular and neurological disorders.

Understanding the science of aging requires investigating the consequences of inflammation. Low-grade, chronic inflammation, or "inflammaging," characterizes aging. Inflammatory processes, which are intimately linked to the immune system's response to stress and cellular damage, influence age-related disorders.

Factors Affecting Longevity

Although DNA certainly contributes to our potential lifetime, research indicates that environmental factors and lifestyle choices have a significant influence on longevity. Analyzing these characteristics provides valuable insight into how people might improve their chances of living longer, healthier lives.

Genetics and Longevity:

By discovering genetic markers linked with extreme lifespan, research on centenarians and their families helps us understand the genetic component of longevity. Although hereditary variables account for 20-30% of human lifetime variance, lifestyle decisions can alter how particular genes are expressed.

Lifestyle Choices:

Longevity has traditionally been linked to good lifestyle choices including modest alcohol use, no smoking, and regular physical activity. Exercise, for example, increases mitochondrial function, preserves cardiovascular health, and promotes overall well-being.

Social and Environmental Factors:

To live a long and healthy life, it is necessary to have both a supportive environment and meaningful social ties. It has been shown via research that people who have extensive social networks often live for a longer period, which highlights the value of maintaining positive mental health and meaningful interactions. In addition to this, the effect of environmental factors such as access to green areas and the quality of the air cannot be ignored since it is impossible to do so.

The Role of Nutrition in Aging

Nutrition emerges as a major factor that, depending on how it is managed, may either speed up or slow down the aging process as researchers unravel the intricate web of factors that influence longevity. Our meal includes the foundational components necessary for the generation of energy, the repair of damaged cells, and the upkeep of overall health.

Nutrient-Rich Foods:

Minerals and vitamins that are necessary play a significant role in a variety of bodily processes. Fruits, vegetables, whole grains, and lean cuts of meat are examples of foods that are rich in nutrients and provide the body with the resources it needs to function at its highest potential. For instance, antioxidants, which can be found in great quantities in brightly colored fruits and vegetables, have a role in the mitigation of oxidative stress and the repair of damaged cells.

Hydration and Longevity:

It is crucial to a diet that promotes lifespan to keep a sufficient amount of water, even though this fact is commonly overlooked. Water is essential for all of the biological activities, including the removal of waste products and the processes that take place in the cells. The overall amount of fluid ingested is increased by beverages such as herbal teas and other liquids that are hydrating.

CHAPTER 1: THE BASICS OF AN EXTENDED LIFE DIET

Starting on the path to longer lifespans requires making dietary choices that actively support the body's ability to fend against aging while also providing food. This level entails making dietary decisions that will lay a solid foundation. We explore the importance of nutrient-dense meals and the specific ingredients that make them up, such as the essential vitamins, minerals, and antioxidants, as well as their function in scavenging free radicals, in this discussion of the foundations of a diet that encourages longevity.

Nutrient-Rich Foods

A diet that focuses on extending life should revolve around foods that are high in nutrients and give the body the elements and nutrients it needs to function at its optimum. These foods provide an abundance of vitamins, minerals, and other bioactive components that support an individual's overall health in addition to providing the energy required for daily activities.

Essential Vitamins and Minerals

- **_Vitamins:_**

Important vitamins are organic compounds that are essential to several physiological processes. They support the maintenance of healthy skin, vision, and other body systems. They also aid in the functioning of the immune system and act as cofactors in enzyme activities. For long-term health, eating a variety of foods strong in vitamins is crucial.

- **Vitamin A:** For good skin, vision, and immune system function, vitamin A is necessary. Leafy greens, liver, and orange and yellow veggies all contain it.

- **Vitamin C:** Bell peppers, berries, and citrus fruits are rich sources of vitamin C, a potent antioxidant that supports the immune system and collagen synthesis.

- **Vitamin D:** Good sources of vitamin D include fortified dairy products, fatty fish, and exposure to sunlight. Vitamin D is essential for strong bones and a functioning immune system.

- **Vitamin E:** Nuts, seeds, and spinach all contain vitamin E, an antioxidant that helps protect cells from oxidative damage.

- **Vitamin K:** Soybeans, leafy green vegetables, and broccoli are rich sources of vitamin K, which is required for blood clotting and strong bones.

- **Minerals:**

Inorganic elements known as essential minerals are necessary for a wide range of physiological functions, including bone health and nerve transmission.

- **Calcium:** The body absorbs more calcium when it consumes dairy products, leafy greens, and fortified meals, which helps maintain strong bones and muscles.

- **Iron:** Iron is essential for the synthesis of all energy and for the delivery of oxygen. It may be found in red meat, lentils, and dark leafy vegetables.

- **Magnesium:** This mineral, which is present in whole grains, nuts, seeds, and leafy greens, promotes the function of the muscles and nerves.

- **Potassium:** is a mineral found in potatoes, bananas, and leafy greens that is vital for heart health and blood pressure management.

- **Zinc:** Zinc, which is included in meats, dairy products, and legumes, is crucial for the immune system's operation and the

healing of wounds.

Antioxidants and Free Radicals

Antioxidants are essential for combating free radicals, which are unstable chemicals produced by regular cellular functions and in reaction to environmental stressors like pollution and ultraviolet light. Free radicals can harm cells, which accelerates aging and several chronic illnesses. One of the most important ways to lessen the effects of free radicals is to include foods high in antioxidants in your diet.

Sources of Antioxidants:

- **Berries:** Strawberries, raspberries, and blueberries are rich in anthocyanins and quercetin, two powerful antioxidants that may help protect against oxidative stress.

- **Dark Chocolate:** Strawberries, raspberries, and blueberries are rich in anthocyanins and quercetin, two powerful antioxidants that may help protect against oxidative stress.

- **Nuts and Seeds:** Almonds, walnuts, and sunflower seeds are rich in vitamin E, selenium, and other antioxidants that enhance cellular defense.

- **Colorful Vegetables:** Vegetables such as tomatoes, spinach, and bell peppers are rich in antioxidants, including lutein, beta-carotene, and lycopene.

- **Green Tea:** Green tea has a high catechin content and is well-known for its anti-inflammatory and antioxidant properties.

Benefits of Antioxidants:

- **Protection of Cells:** Antioxidants neutralize free radicals, preventing them from damaging cellular constituents such as proteins, lipids, and DNA.

- **Anti-Inflammatory Effects:** Antioxidants have been shown to reduce inflammation, both acute and chronic, which can be caused by aging and sickness.

- **Heart Health:** Antioxidants may assist in the maintenance of healthy cardiovascular function by reducing oxidative stress and encouraging healthy blood vessel function.

BALANCED MACRONUTRIENTS

A sustainable and healthful diet should aim to achieve equilibrium across the three categories of macronutrients (proteins, fats, and carbs). This is one of the main tenets of a healthy diet that extends a person's life. Every one of these macronutrients has a unique and essential role in supporting a multitude of critical physiological functions, such as sustaining steady energy levels and repairing damaged cells. This comprehensive analysis delves into the importance of preserving a balance between macronutrients and the specific roles that each macronutrient plays in lifespan.

Protein for Cellular Repair

The building blocks of life, proteins are necessary for the development, upkeep, and regulation of almost all cellular functions inside the body. From the biochemical reactions that are aided by enzymes to the immune system protections that antibodies offer, proteins are engaged in a myriad of activities that are critical to leading a long and healthy life. An in-depth analysis of the role that protein plays in maintaining general health and repairing damaged cells may be found below:

Sources of Protein:

- **Animal Sources:** Complete proteins with all of the required amino acids are found in meat, chicken, fish, eggs, and dairy products.

- **Plant Sources:** Legumes, beans, nuts, seeds, and grains are all components of a diet high in protein, even if some amino acids found in animal products might not be found in plant sources.

Benefits of Protein for Longevity:

Cellular Repair: Cellular repair, sometimes referred to as tissue reconstruction, depends on proteins for the effective operation and regeneration of cells.

Maintenance of Muscle: We must eat adequate protein since as we become older, our capacity to maintain muscular mass decreases.

This is particularly important for the older population's overall mobility and strength.

Immune Support: Protein is essential for supporting a healthy immune system and preventing illness since it is the building block of both antibodies and immune system components.

Protein Quality and Quantity:

Full vs. Incomplete Proteins: The vast majority of proteins derived from plant sources are incomplete, but the proteins derived from animal sources are often complete. If you consume a variety of plant-based proteins at different times throughout the day, you may ensure that your amino acid profile will be well-balanced.

Daily Protein Requirements: Protein requirements vary from person to person based on factors such as age, amount of physical activity, and overall health. A healthy diet usually includes sources of protein that account for 10–35 percent of daily calorie consumption.

Brain Function and Healthy Fats

Fats are commonly misunderstood in the context of a healthy diet. While ingesting poor fats in excess can cause a variety of health issues, including cardiovascular disease, having healthy fats in the diet is critical for overall health, particularly brain function.

Sources of Healthy Fats:

- **Monounsaturated fats:** These fats, which are linked to heart health and may have anti-inflammatory properties, can be found in almonds, avocados, and olive oil.

- **Polyunsaturated Fats:** Walnuts, flaxseeds, chia seeds, and fatty fish are high in omega-3 and omega-6 fatty acids, which are essential for brain function (such as mackerel and salmon).

- **Moderate Intake of Saturated Fats:** While taking too much-saturated fat—found in animal products and some tropical oils—can be detrimental, integrating saturated fats in a balanced diet requires moderation.

The Function of Fats in the Brain:

- **Structural Component:** Because the brain is typically 60% fat, fatty acids, particularly omega-3s, are crucial for maintaining the structural integrity of brain cells.

- **Production of Neurotransmitters:** Neurotransmitters are chemical messengers that facilitate communication between nerve cells. Fats play a part in their creation. This is necessary to preserve overall mental health, cognitive function, and mood stability.

- **Insulation and Protection:** Fats encase and protect nerve cells, performing the function of an insulator to speed up the transmission of electrical impulses in the brain.

Balancing Fats for Longevity:

The amount of omega-3 fatty acids relative to omega-6: Establishing a healthy equilibrium between these two fatty acids is of the utmost importance. Even while both are essential, inflammation may be the result of an imbalance that is skewed toward omega-6 fatty acids, which is typical of diets in Western countries.

Carbohydrates for Long-Lasting Energy

Carbohydrates are the primary source of energy that the body utilizes to fuel a variety of physiological processes, such as the contraction of muscles, activity in the brain, and the breakdown of cellular material. However, the kind of carbohydrates and the quality of those carbohydrates that are consumed have a significant impact on both health and lifespan.

Types of Carbohydrates:

- **Complex Carbohydrates:** Complex carbs included in whole grains, vegetables, legumes, and fruits give sustained energy due to their delayed digestion and glucose release.

- **Simple Carbohydrates:** Simple carbs are sugars that induce rapid fluctuations in blood sugar levels. They can be found in processed meals, candy, and sugary beverages.

Carbohydrates' Function in Longevity:

- **Brain Function:** Glucose is the brain's primary energy source. Consuming complex carbohydrates ensures a steady supply of glucose, which aids attention and cognitive performance.

- **Physical Endurance:** Carbohydrates are required for endurance and peak performance in those who participate in physical exercise regularly. While exercising, muscles use glycogen, which is stored glucose, as a significant source of energy.

- **Digestive Health:** Dietary fiber is a key component of complex carbohydrates. It promotes satiety, regulates bowel movements, and supports a healthy gut flora.

Choosing Quality Carbohydrates:

- **Whole Grains:** Whole wheat products, quinoa, brown rice, and oats include complex carbohydrates, fiber, vitamins, and minerals.

- **Vibrant Fruits and Vegetables:** In addition to carbs, they give a multitude of antioxidants, vitamins, and minerals that are needed for optimum health.

- **Reducing Sugar Intake:** Reducing the quantity of added sugars in processed foods is critical for preventing blood sugar imbalances and related health concerns.

CHAPTER 2: THE INFLUENCE OF EATING ONLY PLANTS

Lately, there has been a lot of focus placed on the need to consume a diet that is mostly made up of foods derived from plants to maximize one's chances of living a long and healthy life. Diets that are mostly composed of plant foods emphasize consuming plants in their whole, unprocessed forms as much as possible while minimizing or excluding the intake of foods derived from animals. This chapter analyzes the benefits of sticking to a plant-based diet by delving into the advantages of adopting a plant-forward approach, eating a variety of vegetables, and realizing the relevance of consuming whole grains and fiber for maintaining good gastrointestinal function.

The Plant-Forward Approach

A plant-forward diet should not be confused with a vegan or vegetarian diet in its purest form. Instead, it encourages individuals to put more of an emphasis on consuming meals that come from plants, even while they are free to still consume animal products if they so desire. This flexible approach creates the framework for a diversified, nutrient-rich diet, which has been linked to a range of different health benefits.

The Advantages of a Plant-Based Diet

Cardiovascular Health:

- **Lower Risk of Heart Disease:** Plant-based diets have been linked to a decreased risk of heart disease because they lower blood pressure, and cholesterol, and enhance vascular health.

- **Effects of Antioxidants and Anti-Inflammatory Foods:** Antioxidant-rich foods promote cardiovascular health by lowering inflammation and oxidative stress.

Weight Management:

- **Encouragement of a Healthy Weight:** Plant-based diets are naturally lower in calories and saturated fats, making them excellent for weight control and reducing obesity-related disorders.

- **High Content of Fiber:** Plant-based meals with high fiber content keep people satisfied for longer, encouraging satiety and lowering overall calorie consumption.

Metabolic Health:

- **Increased Sensitivity to Insulin:** A plant-based diet may improve insulin sensitivity, lowering the risk of type 2 diabetes.
- **Control of Blood Sugar Levels:** Stable blood sugar levels are necessary for metabolic health, and complex carbohydrates included in plant-based diets help with this.

Cancer Prevention:

- **Anticancer Properties:** Several plant compounds, including antioxidants and phytochemicals, have demonstrated anti-cancer activity. This may help to lower the likelihood of developing certain types of cancer.

- **Fiber and Digestive Health:** A fiber-rich diet can help maintain a healthy digestive tract and reduce the risk of colon cancer.

Longevity and Overall Health:

- **Decreased Inflammation:** Diets that are high in plants contain natural anti-inflammatory characteristics, which may help lessen the chronic inflammation that is caused by aging and the diseases that are associated with aging.

- **Rich in Nutrients:** The great variety of plant foods available ensures that the body receives a sufficient amount of essential vitamins, minerals, and phytonutrients, hence enhancing overall health and extending lifespan.

A Rainbow of Vegetables Included

The vibrant colors of fruits and vegetables represent a variety of nutrients, each of which has a unique impact on health. You can be sure you're getting a range of vital antioxidants, minerals, vitamins, and phytochemicals when you eat a rainbow of veggies.

Colorful Antioxidants:

- **Beta-carotene:** Beta-carotene, a precursor to vitamin A, is present in orange and yellow foods such as carrots and sweet potatoes. Both the immune system and vision are supported by it.

- **Lycopene:** Lycopene, which is abundant in tomatoes, watermelon, and pink grapefruit, has been connected to a lower risk of heart disease and several cancers.

- **Flavonoids:** Flavonoids are antioxidants and anti-inflammatory compounds that are present in a wide variety of fruits and vegetables.

Cruciferous Vegetables:

- Vegetables strong in glucosinolates, which may have anti-cancer effects, include broccoli, cauliflower, and kale.

- Sulforaphane: Studies have been conducted on the potential of sulforaphane to aid in detoxifying and reducing inflammation. Cruciferous veggies contain it.

Leafy Greens:

- Swiss chard, spinach, and kale are examples of leafy greens that are high in vitamins, minerals, and phytonutrients that support overall health and well-being.

- Folate: Richly present in leafy greens, folate is necessary for the synthesis and repair of DNA.

Diversity for Gut Health:

- Vegetables High in Fiber: A range of vegetables provide dietary fiber in different forms, which are vital for maintaining a balanced gut flora.

- Prebiotics: Certain vegetables have a probiotic effect, which promotes the development of beneficial bacteria in the

stomach.

Fiber and Whole Grains for Digestive Health

When consumed as part of a plant-based diet, whole grains not only supply the body with the nutrients it requires but also the dietary fiber that is critical to the digestive tract's continued good health. This contributes to an even greater improvement in the diet's overall nutritional composition.

Whole Grains for Longevity:

- Whole grains, such as barley, quinoa, and brown rice, are an excellent source of a wide range of nutrients, including minerals, antioxidants, and B vitamins.

- Complex Carbs Whole grains include complex carbohydrates, which improve overall vitality by providing energy that lasts for a longer period.

Fiber and Gut Microbiota:

- Sources of Dietary Fiber Whole grains, legumes, fruits, and vegetables are good sources of the dietary fiber that is necessary for maintaining a healthy gut.

- Increased Immunological Response and Decreased Inflammation Associated with Diverse Gut Microbiota Eating a diet that is rich in diversity and well-balanced encourages the growth of a diverse gut microbiota, which has been linked to increased immune system response and decreased inflammation.

Promoting Regular Bowel Movements:

Consuming a sufficient quantity of fiber from whole grains will help you maintain regular bowel movements, which in turn helps promote digestive health and prevent constipation.

A High-Fiber Diet Has Been Linked to a Lower Risk of Colorectal Cancer and Other Digestive Issues Diets high in fiber have been linked to a lower risk of colorectal cancer and other digestive issues.

CHAPTER 3: OPTIMAL HYDRATION

It is hard to overstate the significance of adequate hydration in terms of preserving one's health and adding years to one's life. Water, the elixir of life, is required for the proper functioning of all body systems as well as individual cells. This inquiry into the optimal amount of hydration investigates the advantages of herbal teas and infusions, the role that hydration plays in the operation of cells, the relevance of water for longevity, and the beverages that need to be avoided for long-term health and wellness.

Water and Longevity

Fluid Balance and Homeostasis:

Water is essential for maintaining the equilibrium of body fluids, which in turn supports several physiological processes such as the removal of waste, the regulation of temperature, and the transfer of nutrition. Water also plays an important role in the processes that are carried out by the body.

Homeostasis: The ability of the body to govern its internal environment in response to changes in the environment outside of the body is dependent on proper hydration for both achieving and maintaining homeostasis.

Hydration Is Essential for Cell Function

Cellular Processes and Water:

- Cellular respiration, the mechanism by which cells convert nutrients into energy, depends on water. Effective cellular respiration supports overall metabolic function.

- Transport of Nutrients: Water facilitates the entry of nutrients into cells and the departure of waste products, allowing for optimal cellular function.

- Temperature Regulation: Water helps regulate body temperature by promoting perspiration, which prevents people from being too hot or too tired when exercising.

Hydration and Cognitive Function:

- **Effect on Cognitive Performance:** Research has indicated a link between dehydration and cognitive impairments, including problems with mood, memory, and concentration.

- **Brain Health:** Adequate hydration improves emotional stability and cognitive function, which in turn supports mental health in general.

Joint and Muscle Health:

- **Shock Absorption and Lubrication:** The synovial fluid that lubricates and cushions joints must include water. Staying well-hydrated is crucial for maintaining healthy joints and preventing stiffness.

- **Muscle Efficiency:** Hydrated muscles perform better, reducing the likelihood of cramping and increasing physical output.

Herbal Teas and Infusions

Hydration Beyond Water:

- Hydration from Herbal Infusions and Teas Along with the Numerous Other Health Benefits They Offer, Herbal Infusions and Teas Also Help with General Hydration.

- Antioxidant Content Many different kinds of herbal tea include antioxidants, which are substances that shield cells from the damaging effects of oxidative stress.

- Teas made from herbs with soothing properties, such as chamomile and lavender, can assist individuals in relaxing and better coping with the effects of stress.

Popular Herbal Teas:

- Peppermint Tea is a tea that does not include caffeine and is recognized for its ability to moisturize and refresh the palate. It is also known for its ability to aid digestion.

- Ginger Tea: Ginger tea, which is well known for its ability to reduce inflammation, also helps digestion and has a warming effect on the body.

- Hibiscus Tea: Because it is rich in antioxidants, hibiscus tea may help enhance hydration levels as well as the health of the cardiovascular system.

- Green Tea: Even though it includes caffeine, green tea is an excellent hydrator and has other health benefits as well, including an increased metabolic rate and improved cognitive function.

Infusions and Fruit-Infused Water:

Infusions of Fruits and Herbs Adding cucumber, fruit, or herb slices to water gives it a more flavorful profile and encourages consumers to consume more water overall.

Electrolytes that occur naturally Citrus fruit infusions, such as those produced with lemons and oranges, are a good source of electrolytes that exist naturally and help maintain mineral balance while also promoting hydration.

Beverages to Avoid

The Dangers of Dehydrating Drinks:

Sugary Drinks and Aging:

- Empty Calories: Sugary drinks with added sugar, such as fruit juices and sodas, offer empty calories that can contribute to weight gain and obesity.

- Long-term inflammation brought on by excessive sugar consumption has been linked to accelerated aging and age-related diseases.

- Glycation: The process through which carbohydrates bind to proteins to produce AGEs (advanced glycation end products) is known to be associated with aging. Sugars may have a role in this procedure.

Limiting Alcohol for Longevity:

- **Dehydration:** Alcohol can induce fluid loss and dehydration as it is a diuretic and increases the output of urine.

- **Liver Health:** The liver is a vital organ for overall health and detoxification, and drinking too much alcohol can impair liver function.

- **Effects on the Brain:** Long-term and excessive alcohol use is associated with an increased risk of neurodegenerative diseases and cognitive decline.

Balancing Choices for Optimal Hydration:

The Crucial Role of Moderation Treating yourself once in a while is fine, even if it is recommended that you stay away from alcoholic beverages and beverages that are high in sugar. Consumption should be done with moderation and consideration to achieve a healthy balance when it comes to hydration.

Water, serves as the Primary Resource The most effective and all-natural method of hydration is the consumption of still water. It does not contribute any calories to the diet, is essential for the activity of cells, and improves overall health.

CHAPTER 4: MINDFUL EATING TECHNIQUES

People who are interested in living a long life and improving their overall health may find that incorporating more mindful eating habits into their diet is an approach that may be both transformative and powerful. This chapter explores the profound connection that exists between the mind and the digestive tract, as well as the role that mindful eating plays in fostering the health of the digestive tract, the strategies that can be used to combat emotional eating, and the fundamentals of intuitive eating, which can lead to a life that is more vibrant and fulfilling.

The Connection Between Mind and Gut

Holistic Approach to Health:

The Connection Between the Brain and the Intestines One of the most fascinating elements of human physiology is the intricate connection that occurs between the brain and the digestive tract. The digestive system and the central nervous system are connected by a communication pathway known as the gut-brain axis. This pathway allows for communication to occur in both ways. The comprehensive quality of our whole health is brought into sharper focus by this technique.

Mindful Eating for Digestive Health

Conscious Consumption:

Consuming mindfully means reducing the speed at which one consumes food, which helps individuals to savor each bite and take in all of the flavor and texture characteristics of the food that they are eating.

The process of chewing and digesting: By breaking down food into smaller pieces and increasing the production of digestive enzymes, vigorous chewing of food is beneficial to the digestive process. This takes place when food is broken down into smaller pieces when chewing.

Strategies for Mindful Eating:

Including the Senses: Including the senses in the dining experience may be achieved by focusing on the meal's color, texture, and aroma. The overall dining experience will be enhanced by this.

Removing Interruptions People are better able to focus on the process of eating and the feelings associated with it when they can avoid or minimize distractions, such as work-related duties or technological gadgets.

Benefits for Digestive Health:

By raising awareness of hunger and fullness cues, mindful eating lowers the risk of overindulging and facilitates the growth of a healthy, balanced relationship with food.

Increased Absorption of Nutrients Improved chewing and digestion help the body absorb more nutrients, which guarantees that the body gets all the essential components from the food it eats.

Emotional Eating Techniques

Understanding Emotional Eating:

Emotional Triggers: Some of the emotional triggers that can lead to binge eating or other kinds of emotional eating are stress, boredom, and melancholy. The first thing that needs to be done to conquer emotional eating is to simply become conscious of the triggers that start it off.

Increasing One's Level of Consciousness To begin cultivating mindful awareness of one's emotional signals and learning to differentiate between physical hunger and emotional cravings, one must first establish conscious awareness of one's emotional cues.

Coping Strategies:

Individuals who practice mindful breathing might learn to pause and assess their emotional state before reaching for food as a source of comfort, which can help them avoid overeating. Because of this, there is a decreased possibility that they may resort to food.

Encourage the discovery of other methods of coping, such as engaging in physical exercise, practicing mindfulness meditation, or reaching out to people to obtain social support.

Developing a Conscious Connection with Food:

Food as Nourishment: By changing one's perspective on food from that of a source of emotional comfort to that of a source of nourishment, one may promote a healthy connection with food.

Acceptance and Self-Compassion: When people adopt an attitude of acceptance and self-compassion, they may deal with emotional problems without turning to destructive eating habits.

Intuitive Eating for Longevity

Accepting Your Intuitive Eating:

A Sensitivity Test for Cues of Hunger and Satiety: The secret to intuitive eating is understanding the signals your body sends out to let you know when you are hungry and full. If people are aware of these signs and pay attention to them, they can eat in a way that is compatible with their physiological needs.

Rejecting Traditional Diets' Restrictive Attitude The restricted mentality of conventional diets is opposed by intuitive eating, which emphasizes a flexible and balanced approach to eating.

Mindful Meal Planning:

Identifying and honoring preferences, intuitive eating recognizes that any food may have a place in a well-balanced, pleasurable diet. One of the most important aspects of intuitive eating is recognizing and respecting desires.

Pleasure and Satisfaction: Putting pleasure and satisfaction on equal footing when meal planning will help you have a better overall eating experience and establish a healthy connection with food.

Principles of Intuitive Eating:

Rejecting the Diet Mentality: Freeing oneself from the restrictive dieting cycle is one of the core tenets of intuitive eating. It necessitates embracing internal cues and letting go of externally imposed norms.

Honoring the Body's Natural Indications of Hunger and Fullness: Paying attention to the body's cues about hunger and fullness may help you make better eating choices and promote a more sustainable and well-rounded approach to getting your nutrition.

Making peace with food and giving everyone permission to eat everything without feeling bad or criticized can lead to a healthier relationship with food and reduce the attractiveness of off-limits things.

Arriving at Contentment Two strategies to enhance the quality of the time spent eating is to be aware of the many feelings that arise and to choose meals that satisfy certain requirements.

Different Approaches to Handling Emotions Creating substitute coping strategies for emotional problems contributes to a more considered and balanced approach to mental health. "Coping with emotions without eating" is one such strategy.

CHAPTER 5: DIETARY TECHNIQUES FOR RESTORING CELLS

The procedures of repairing damaged cells and allowing them to create new ones are complex, but maintaining good health over a long period and living a complete life require both of these things to happen. This investigation into nutritional strategies for cellular repair delves into specific foods that encourage cell regeneration, the role that omega-3 fatty acids play in cellular health, the influence that phytonutrients have on the function of cells, as well as the intriguing ideas of autophagy and fasting.

Foods that Support Cell Regeneration

Essential Nutrients for Cellular Health:

- **Macro and Micronutrients:** A diverse spectrum of nutrients is required for the upkeep, growth, and repair of cellular structures. Consuming the appropriate amounts of macronutrients (carbohydrates, proteins, and fats) and micronutrients is essential to maintaining cellular health (vitamins and minerals).

- **Antioxidants:** Antioxidants protect cells against oxidative stress, which is one of the primary factors in the aging process and the destruction of cells. Consuming meals high in antioxidants is necessary to stimulate the regeneration of cells.

Role of Omega-3 Fatty Acids

Omega-3s and Cellular Membranes:

The capacity of omega-3 fatty acids to create key components of cell membranes is what gives them their structural significance. In particular, eicosapentaenoic acid (EPA) and docosahexaenoic acid (DHA) are two of these components (DHA). They allow membranes to maintain their elasticity, fluidity, and functional capacity.

The anti-inflammatory effects of omega-3 fatty acids are achieved by a reduction in the production of inflammatory molecules and the promotion of an environment that is conducive to cellular repair.

Sources of Omega-3 Fatty Acids:

Salmon, mackerel, and sardines are examples of fatty fish that are high in omega-3 fatty acids.

Both chia seeds and flaxseeds are good plant-based sources of alpha-linolenic acid (ALA), which is a component of EPA and DHA. Chia seeds are especially rich in ALA.

Walnuts: Walnuts, which are rich in ALA, help you ingest more omega-3 fatty acids because of their content.

Balancing Omega-3 to Omega-6 Ratio:

Omega-6 Fatty Acids: Although they are essential, an imbalance in the ratio of omega-3 to omega-6 fatty acids, which is typical of diets consumed in Western countries, may be one of the factors that contribute to inflammation. Fatty acids need to be in a state of equilibrium for cells to perform their functions correctly.

Phytonutrients and Cellular Health

Diverse Plant Compounds:

The function of phytonutrients Phytonutrients, also known as phytochemicals, are bioactive molecules that are found in plants. Phytonutrients play an important role in plant health. They do so in a variety of ways that are beneficial to the health of the cells.

Numerous phytonutrients, such as carotenoids and flavonoids, can act as antioxidants and protect cells from the damage that may be caused by oxidation.

Colorful Fruits and Vegetables:

- Berries: Due to the high anthocyanin content, berries have been shown to have both anti-inflammatory and antioxidant effects.

- Kale, spinach, and Swiss chard are examples of leafy greens that are particularly high in the antioxidants lutein and zeaxanthin, which are beneficial to eye health and cellular defense.

- Tomatoes: The lycopene found in tomatoes has been connected to a reduction in the amount of cellular damage and oxidative stress that the body experiences.

Cruciferous Vegetables and Sulforaphane:

Vegetables such as Brussels sprouts, kale, and broccoli have a high amount of sulforaphane. Sulforaphane is a phytonutrient that may assist with the detoxification of cells and may even have anti-cancer benefits.

Autophagy and Fasting

- Autophagy: The Cell Recycling Process: Definition and Importance Autophagy is a biological process that includes the removal and recycling of damaged or dysfunctional cell components. It is a critical mechanism for maintaining cell integrity and preventing the accumulation of cell debris.

- Lifespan Function: Autophagy has been linked to longevity and a decreased prevalence of age-related diseases. It allows cells to adapt to stress, improving both their survival and functioning.

Intermittent Fasting Protocols

Introduction to Intermittent Fasting:

Intervals of Fasting: In intermittent fasting, periods of eating and fasting are alternated. Common protocols include the 16/8 technique (16 hours of fasting and an 8-hour eating window) and the 5:2 plan (regular eating for five days and reduced calorie intake for two non-consecutive days).

Cellular Adaptations: When fasting, the body uses energy differently. Cells discover alternative sources of energy when there is less glucose available, which promotes autophagy and cellular repair.

Benefits for Cellular Health:

Launching of the Autophagy Process It is common knowledge that intermittent fasting can stimulate autophagy, which in turn enhances the process of cellular recycling and cleansing.

It has been demonstrated that fasting increases the activity of mitochondria, which is significant given that mitochondria are the organelles in cells that are responsible for producing energy. It is essential for the continued existence of a cell's mitochondria that they be in excellent condition.

Fasting-Mimicking Diets

Fasting-Mimicking Diets (FMD):

The Fasting Mimicking Diet (FMD) consists of alternating cycles of a diet that replicate the effects of fasting while still providing certain nutrients. The FMD is defined in this way, and this is the principle behind it. This tactic is meant to enhance the health benefits of fasting without subjecting folks to an absolute denial of their ability to consume any food or drink at all.

Regeneration of Cells A time of FMD It has been discovered that FMD is associated with enhanced autophagy and cellular repair, the outcomes of which are analogous to those that are seen during conventional fasting.

Elements of Diets That Simulate Fasting:

Periods of Low-Calorie Consumption: The FMD usually consists of many days of consuming few calories, sometimes emphasizing plant-based foods as the main source of nourishment.

Composition of Nutrients: Despite the restricted caloric intake, the FMD aims to supply essential nutrients to sustain appropriate cellular function and prevent nutrient deficiencies.

Research and Potential Benefits:

Cellular Regeneration: Several research suggest that FMD may enhance aging indicators, promote cellular regeneration, and improve overall health.

It has been demonstrated that FMD may improve insulin sensitivity and lower the risk factors for age-related illnesses, among other metabolic health advantages. It has been established that FMD and these metabolic advantages are related.

CHAPTER 6: NUTRITIONAL HORMONAL BALANCE

Obtaining hormonal harmony is not the same as just preserving hormonal balance; rather, nourishing the body at the hormonal level is required to sustain its vitality throughout time. This is a necessary component in the pursuit of a long life and total well-being. This inquiry into obtaining hormonal harmony through nutrition delves into the importance of hormonal balance, the impact of diet on hormonal health, foods that promote endocrine function, and the complicated connections that exist between the stomach, the brain, and hormones.

Balancing Hormones for Longevity

Essence of Hormonal Balance:

In addition to their function as messengers, hormones also serve a regulatory role in the body by helping to coordinate a wide range of physiological activities. The control of metabolic processes, as well as growth and reproductive activities, are included in these processes.

Influence on the Length of Life If you want to live a longer life and lower your chances of acquiring age-related health problems, one of the most essential things you can do is strike a healthy balance between your hormones and make sure it stays that way.

Dietary Influence on Hormonal Health

Influence of Nutrients on Hormones:

Hormone Synthesis and Regulation Requirements A healthy, well-balanced diet will contain all of the elements required for hormone production and control.

Fatty Acids and Hormones: Good fats, such as omega-3 fatty acids, are necessary for hormone production, but an unhealthy fat imbalance can disrupt hormonal equilibrium.

Foods and Hormonal Modulation:

Vegetables With Crucial Roles chemicals that aid in the breakdown of estrogen and contribute to hormonal balance may be found in cruciferous vegetables such as broccoli, cabbage, and Brussels sprouts, among other cruciferous vegetables.

Unprocessed Grains: Whole grains, which are high in fiber and also impact insulin and cortisol regulation, can be used to help control blood sugar levels and stabilize them.

Proteins That Are Not High in Fat Both the synthesis of growth hormone and the assistance in the maintenance of muscle mass are required for the preservation of hormonal homeostasis. Protein-rich foods help stimulate the production of growth hormones and aid in the maintenance of muscle mass.

Foods that Promote Hormonal Balance

Nutrient-Rich Choices:

Iodine-Rich Foods: Iodine is essential for thyroid function. Seaweed, fish, and iodized salt are good iodine sources.

Foods High in Zinc: The production of sex hormones requires zinc. Foods high in zinc include oysters, pumpkin seeds, and lentils.

Sources of Vitamin D: Meals high in vitamin D, such as fatty fish and fortified dairy products, and sun exposure both have an impact on hormone regulation.

Adaptogenic Herbs:

Ashwagandha: Known for its adaptogenic properties, ashwagandha controls stress hormones including cortisol, which may help maintain hormonal balance.

Rhodiola: Known to reduce cortisol levels, this plant may help regulate hormone imbalances brought on by stress.

The Hormone-Gut-Brain Connection

Complex Interplay Between Systems:

The microbiota that live in one's gut. The bacteria that dwell in the gut number in the billions, and they are responsible for regulating not just hormonal signals but also the digestive process, the absorption of nutrients, and the regulation of hormonal signals.

The gut-brain axis refers to the two-way communication that takes place between the digestive tract and the brain. This communication has an impact not only on the hormone production process but also on the overall physiological homeostasis.

Probiotics and Hormonal Balance

Role of Probiotics:

Beneficial bacteria known as probiotics play an important role in maintaining a healthy gut microbiota, which in turn affects hormone synthesis. They may affect the axis between the stomach and the brain, which would then have ramifications for the production and regulation of hormones.

foods that have undergone the process of fermentation Probiotics are beneficial bacteria that are found in foods like yogurt, kefir, sauerkraut, and kimchi. These bacteria help keep the digestive tract healthy and may even improve hormonal equilibrium.

Specific Hormonal Impact:

- Estrogen Metabolism: The use of some probiotics may play a part in the promotion of the metabolism of estrogen, which in turn may lower the risk of developing hormonal disorders. Live bacteria that are native to the digestive tract are known as probiotics.

- Regulation of Cortisol: The microbiota in the gut can have an effect on levels of cortisol, which in turn can affect how the body reacts to stress and how well it maintains hormonal balance.

Prebiotics for Gut Health

Beneficial gut bacteria are given a food supply when prebiotics, which are fibers that cannot be digested, are consumed. This, in turn, enhances the bacteria's ability to reproduce and increases their overall activity levels.

Foods like garlic, onions, leeks, bananas, and asparagus all have a high concentration of prebiotic fibers in their composition.

Impact on Hormonal Harmony:

Short-Chain Fatty Acids (SCFAs): Short-Chain Fatty Acids are formed when the bacteria in the stomach digest prebiotics. These SCFAs are beneficial to the body. SCFAS may have a positive impact on the regulation of hormones.

Insulin Sensitivity: There is some evidence to suggest that prebiotics have a role in enhanced insulin sensitivity. Prebiotics may be found in foods like yogurt and fermented vegetables. Because of this, there is a possibility that the hormonal balance may be affected, in particular about metabolic health.

CHAPTER 7: ANTI-INFLAMMATORY EATING

Anti-inflammatory diet is one of the best nutritional strategies for long-term health and well-being. An anti-inflammatory diet may help people reduce inflammation and improve their overall health, as chronic inflammation has been linked to several age-related diseases. This study on anti-inflammatory eating looks at the connection between aging and chronic inflammation, enumerates items to avoid, discusses anti-inflammatory foods, and examines the vital role that herbs and spices play in creating delectable, anti-inflammatory dishes.

Chronic Inflammation and Aging

Understanding the Connection:

The body uses inflammation as a protective mechanism, and it is a natural and essential part of that defense. On the other hand, chronic inflammation can speed up aging and contribute to the development of several illnesses.

The Impact of Aging on Inflammation An ongoing, low-grade condition of inflammation that is commonly referred to as "inflammation" can be brought on by the aging process itself. Increased inflammation has been connected to some diseases, such as metabolic dysfunction, neurological problems, and cardiovascular disease.

Inflammatory Foods to Avoid

Proinflammatory Culprits:

Foods that have been refined and processed Processed and refined meals such as sugary snacks, pastries, and white bread are examples of processed and refined foods that can cause inflammation.

It is advised to avoid meals containing artificial trans fats because research has proven that these fats induce inflammation and are hence prevalent in some processed and fried foods.

Excess Omega-6 Fatty Acids Cause Inflammation While omega-6 fatty acids are essential, an imbalance with omega-3 fatty acids can cause inflammation. Some vegetable oils, such as corn and soybean oil, are listed as sources.

Added Sugars and Sweetened Beverages:

A high intake of added sugars, which are commonly found in sugary beverages and desserts, has been linked to elevated levels of inflammatory markers. This might have a function in inflammation.

Insulin Deficiency Insulin resistance is a condition associated with inflammation and several metabolic disorders. Excess sugar consumption has been linked to insulin resistance.

Processed Meats and Red Meat:

Nitrites and Nitrates: Nitrites and nitrates are inflammatory chemicals. Nitrites and nitrates are commonly found in processed meats.

Saturated Fats: A high intake of saturated fats, particularly those produced from red and processed meats, has been associated with inflammation and an increased risk of developing chronic illnesses.

Incorporating Anti-Inflammatory Foods

Embracing an Anti-Inflammatory Plate:

- Fruits and vegetables are high in phytochemicals and antioxidants, which help reduce inflammation. Cruciferous vegetables, leafy greens, and berries are extremely nutritious.

- Fatty fish, such as salmon, mackerel, and sardines, are high in omega-3 fatty acids, which have anti-inflammatory properties.

- Almonds, walnuts, chia seeds, and flaxseeds are high in omega-3 fatty acids and hence aid anti-inflammatory pathways.

- Whole Grains: High-fiber whole grains, such as brown rice and quinoa, help to stabilize blood sugar levels and may have anti-inflammatory qualities.

Healthy Fats and Oils:

- Extra virgin olive oil contains anti-inflammatory polyphenols as well as monounsaturated fats.

- Avocado: Avocados are high in antioxidants and monounsaturated fats, making them an excellent addition to an anti-inflammatory diet.

Herbs and Spices:

- Turmeric and Curcumin: Turmeric's primary component, curcumin, has powerful anti-inflammatory and antioxidant properties.

- Gingerol: Gingerol is an analgesic and anti-inflammatory chemical.

- Garlic contains the chemical allicin, which has immune-stimulating and anti-inflammatory properties.

The Function of Herbs and Spices

Harnessing the Power of Nature:

The fact that herbs and spices have been employed for hundreds of years not only for their flavor but also for the medical advantages they bring is the primary factor that contributes to the historical relevance of these foods. There are several that have qualities that help lessen inflammation and protect cells from harm caused by free radicals.

Turmeric, Ginger, and Other Powerhouses

Turmeric and Curcumin:

- Curcumin's anti-inflammatory properties are widely known. Curcumin, the main ingredient in turmeric, is widely known for its potent anti-inflammatory properties.

- Enhanced By mixing turmeric with black pepper, which already includes piperine, the bioavailability of curcumin can be improved. This combination increases the body's absorption of curcumin.

Ginger and Gingerol:

Effects: Gingerol, a bioactive component of ginger, has been demonstrated to have anti-inflammatory and antioxidant activities.

Digestive System Advantages: Ginger can improve general health by aiding digestion.

Cinnamon:

Cinnamon includes compounds with anti-inflammatory and antibacterial properties, which are responsible for cinnamon's health benefits.

Cinnamon may also help regulate blood sugar levels, which is another health advantage of this spice.

Rosemary:

Carnosic Acid Content: Carnosic acid, which is found in rosemary, has been studied for its anti-inflammatory and neuroprotective activities.

Rosemary provides flavor to recipes while also providing possible health benefits.

Creating Flavorful, Anti-Inflammatory Meals

Balancing Flavors and Textures:

Oils Infused with Herbs Adding anti-inflammatory elements to meals while increasing their flavor using herb-infused oils, such as rosemary-infused olive oil, is achievable when you manufacture your herb-infused oils.

Herbs that are in season Fresh herbs like cilantro, parsley, and basil not only add taste to dishes, but they also have anti-inflammatory properties.

Spice Blends: Making your spice mixes is a fun way to add diversity and depth of flavor to your cooking. Turmeric, cumin, and coriander are among the anti-inflammatory spices that perform well in spice mixes.

Anti-Inflammatory Recipes:

Golden Smoothie with Turmeric and Ginger: This energizing drink derives its anti-inflammatory and energizing effects from the combination of turmeric, ginger, coconut milk, and just a hint of black pepper. These ingredients create a Golden Smoothie.

Salmon Cooked in the Oven or on the Grill and Seasoned with Fresh Lemon and Dill: Salmon prepared in the oven or on the grill and seasoned with fresh lemon and dill makes for a dish that is not only delicious but also high in omega-3 fatty acids and anti-inflammatory.

Quinoa Salad with Vibrant Vegetables: A quinoa salad that consists of a variety of colorful vegetables, fresh herbs, and a drizzle of olive oil makes for a meal that is full of nutrients and helps to reduce inflammation.

CHAPTER 8: PERSONALIZED LONGEVITY STRATEGIES

When it comes to optimizing one's well-being and meeting one's specific requirements, a strategy that takes the view that "one size fits all" is usually insufficient. Personalized longevity plans, which are built on the evaluation of an individual's needs, genetic influences on nutrition, and tailored diets for particular health goals, provide a nuanced and effective strategy for promoting a vibrant and long-lasting life. These plans are based on the idea that different people have different dietary requirements and genetic make-ups that affect how they respond to certain nutrients. People who follow these programs have a better chance of living healthier lives for longer. This investigation into personalized plans for increasing longevity delves into the complexities of determining an individual's needs, the impact of genetic influences on nutrition, the art of tailoring diets to specific health goals, and the role of longevity-boosting supplements, including essential supplements for aging well as well as the potential risks and benefits associated with the use of these supplements. Ultimately, the goal of this investigation is to develop individualized plans for increasing longevity.

Assessing Individual Needs

Acknowledging Each Person's Individuality:

The concept that every single person contains a unique bio-individuality that is molded by aspects such as their genetics, lifestyle, environment, and medical history is referred to as "bio-individuality." The phrase "bio-individuality" relates to this theory.

It is vital to have a flexible and customized approach to dealing with these problems since the needs of an individual might change over time regarding their nutrition, their level of physical activity, and their general level of well-being.

Genetic Influences on Nutrition

Unraveling the Genetic Code:

Nutrigenomics is the study of how various individual genetic variations influence reactions to nutrition and affect a person's overall health. Nutrigenomics also refers to the study of how different individuals respond differently to certain foods.

Genes that include polymorphisms Polymorphisms, also known as variations in genes, can affect the metabolic process, as well as the body's ability to absorb and use nutrients.

Practical Application:

The MTHFR Gene and Folate Metabolism People who have variations in the MTHFR gene have a higher chance of having an altered folate metabolism. Because of this, it is essential to have a customized folate intake.

Inability to Digest Lactose and Its Connection to the LCT Gene Lactose tolerance can be influenced by genetic variants in the LCT gene, which in turn might affect the demand for dairy products or lactose-free alternatives.

Diets Adapted to Particular Health Objectives

Precision Nutrition:

When it comes to weight management, personalized approaches take into account a variety of characteristics, such as an individual's metabolic rate, body composition, and sensitivity to different food patterns. Personalized approaches also take into account whether or not the individual is trying to lose or maintain their current weight.

Those who are striving to regain control of their health after being diagnosed with a condition such as diabetes or insulin resistance should carefully evaluate how the reactions of their blood sugar levels will be affected by the meals they consume.

Dietary plans that are tailored to an individual's unique health profile can be designed to take into consideration the individual's levels of cholesterol and blood pressure, in addition to other risk factors that contribute to the development of cardiovascular disease.

Flexibility and Sustainability:

Adapting to Preferences: Individual preferences, cultural influences, and lifestyle aspects are taken into consideration by individualized longevity programs to build sustainable eating habits.

Including Restrictions on Diet: People with particular dietary restrictions, such as vegetarianism or gluten sensitivity, benefit from plan designs that take their dietary choices and nutritional needs into consideration.

Longevity-Boosting Supplements

Supplements as a Complement to Nutrition:

Supplements Can Act as a Bridge to Address Nutritional Gaps When it is difficult to meet certain dietary demands via the consumption of food alone, supplements can serve as a bridge to address the nutritional gaps.

Support Directed Toward a Specific Aim Certain dietary supplements aid with overall well-being by treating age-related concerns or by concentrating on achieving specific health goals.

Vital Supplements for Healthy Aging

Foundational Nutrients:

Vitamin D: This is crucial for the immune system and bone health, and it may reduce the risk of chronic illnesses. It's crucial to get enough sun exposure and supplements, especially for older people.

Omega-3 Fatty Acids: Taking omega-3 fatty acid supplements, particularly those made from fish oil, can lower inflammation, improve cognitive function, and promote heart health.

In addition to being necessary for strong bones, magnesium, and calcium are also involved in muscular contraction, nerve transmission, and overall metabolic balance.

***Antioxidants and Anti-Inflammatories:**ingredient*

Potent antioxidants that can slow down aging, such as vitamins C and E, can help fight free radicals.

It is commonly recognized that curcumin, or turmeric extract, has anti-inflammatory properties. Additionally, it could enhance general well-being and joint health.

Resveratrol: One antioxidant that may benefit cardiovascular health is resveratrol. Some fruits and red wine contain it.

***Probiotics for Gut Health:**ingredient*

- **Preserving Gut Microbiota:** Probiotics support immune system development, nutrition absorption, and digestion by assisting in maintaining the proper balance of intestinal microbes in the stomach.

- **Fermented Foods and Pills:** Probiotics support immune system development, nutrition absorption, and digestion by assisting in maintaining the proper balance of intestinal microbes in the stomach.

Potential Risks and Benefits

Balancing Act:

Individual Response: The usefulness of supplements might vary depending on a person's genetics, lifestyle, and overall health.

Monitoring and Modifying: It's important to routinely monitor health markers and consult with medical professionals to adjust supplement regimens in response to changing needs.

Risks and Considerations:

It is essential to perform routine checks on one's health markers and consult with qualified medical professionals to adapt one's supplement regimen in response to shifting requirements.

Bioavailability and Absorption:

Increasing Bioavailability: The bioavailability of several different dietary supplements can be improved via the application of certain formulations or combinations. Absorption can be improved, for instance, by taking vitamin D in conjunction with a healthy source of fat.

Receiving your nutrients from whole foods provides more benefits than getting them from supplements, such as fiber, phytonutrients, and a more complete nutritional profile. Although supplements are more convenient, getting your nutrients from entire foods has more benefits.

CONCLUSION

We have traversed a landscape that is abundant with ideas, strategies, and a celebration of well-being within the vast fabric of a lifespan. As we come to the end of this in-depth exploration of the factors that contribute to longevity, it is becoming abundantly evident that the route to a long and active life is dynamic and unique to each person.

Recognizing Small Wins and Progress Made It is essential to one's longevity to be able to recognize and appreciate one's accomplishments, no matter how insignificant they may seem. These victories—whether they manifest in the form of enhanced well-being, improved eating mindfulness, or enhanced physical fitness—serve as powerful catalysts that encourage people to continue moving forward on their journey. People may develop a momentum that cultivates a feeling of resilience and achievement by monitoring lifespan markers, making feasible goals, and adopting a perspective that values every improvement.

Recognizing That There Is No Short-Cut to Wellness:

Beyond a person's chronological age, longevity may be seen as a commitment to maintaining one's physical and mental health over one's whole life. This way is distinguished by the cultivation of good habits, adaptability in the face of change, and a holistic approach that takes into consideration an individual's physical, mental, and emotional well-being. Accepting failures as opportunities for personal development and seeing tenacity and consistency as the pillars of success are key components in the formation of a resilient mentality that integrates wellness into day-to-day activities.

Key Reflections on the Journey:

Taking into account the extensive path of lifespan leads to significant realizations like:

Understanding the interdependence of the body, mind, and emotions is essential to holistic well-being. Creating a harmonious relationship between these components results in a complete and enduring sense of existence.

The importance of eating mindfully becomes clear as a central subject. A nutrient-rich diet, macronutrient balance, and avoiding pro-inflammatory choices are important tactics for increasing cellular vitality and lifespan.

Customized Methods: Given the unique characteristics of bio-individuality, it is imperative to implement customized wellness strategies. Customization ensures a distinct path to lifespan based on genetics, preferences, and evolving health requirements.

Mobility as Therapeutic Intervention: When exercise is handled with enthusiasm, it may be turned from a chore into a source of vitality. Either via structured exercise or recreational pursuits, contented movement enhances longevity and overall health.

Mindful Practices: It becomes evident that a long life depends on reducing stress. Practicing mindfulness, meditation, and cultivating an optimistic mindset all promote resilience in the face of hardship and mental health.

Lifelong Learning: The commitment to lifelong learning becomes a cornerstone. A long and happy life needs the pursuit of intellectually challenging hobbies, an inquiring spirit, and the joy of self-discovery.

Establishing a Support System: Recognizing the importance of social networks and a supportive community is essential. Supportive, goal-oriented, and well-being-promoting partnerships are vital elements of the long-term path.

www.ingramcontent.com/pod-product-compliance
Lightning Source LLC
Chambersburg PA
CBHW050827260726
48660CB00004B/1643